MGUS, Plasmacytoma and Multiple Myeloma:
Fast Focus Study Guide

JT Thomas, MD

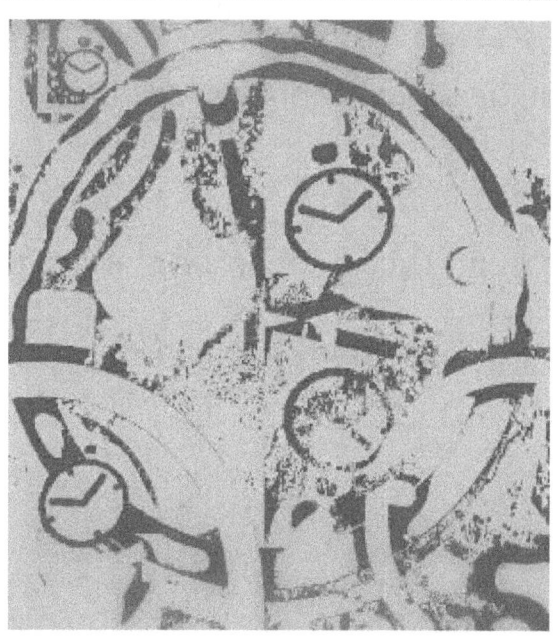

Acknowledgements

I dedicate this book to my beautiful wife and children, who I love more than all the water in all the oceans and all the seas.

CONTENTS

- This book is written to help the reader further understand MGUS, plasmacytoma, and multiple myeloma.

- This book is written in a simple and easy to read format designed for medical students, residents and physicians who are preparing for boards.

- This book simplifies a complicated medical issue so you will remember the important details.

- You will not get caught up in the minutia. Just the facts are found in this book.

- This Fast Focus Study Guide will provide you with a practical review of the key information you need to know.

- Buy this book now if you want this quick and concise information

Monoclonal gammopathy, plasmacytoma and multiple myeloma are diseases that can be categorized as plasma cell dyscrasias.

Plasma cell dyscrasias are characterized by an abnormal proliferation of a monoclonal population of plasma cells.

These diseases are often associated with the production of a monoclonal protein that can be measured with the serum protein electrophoresis (SPEP).

The SPEP uses electrophoresis to expose blood serum to an electric current to separate the serum protein components into five major fractions based on groups of similar size, shape, and charge.

The 5 major fractions identified in serum protein electrophoresis include the serum albumin, alpha-1 globulins, alpha-2 globulins, beta globulins, and gamma globulins.

The 5 major fractions can be placed into a
graph as outlined on the next page.

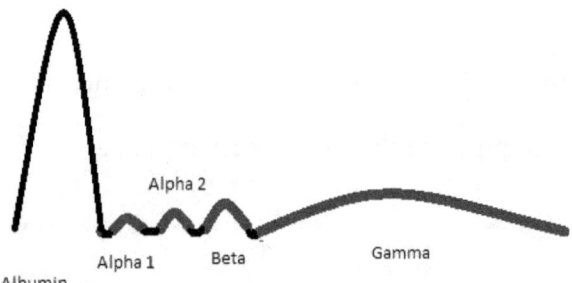

Normal Hemoglobin Electrophoresis

These five major proteins can be defined further.

Albumin

Albumin is the primary protein in the blood and therefore is the largest fraction on the SPEP.

Alpha 1

The Alpha-1 fraction is made up of alpha-1 antitrypsin and thyroid binding globulin.

Alpha 2

The Alpha-2 fraction consists of ceruloplasm and haptoglobin.

Beta 1

The Beta-1 fraction is made up of several proteins
including transferrin.

Gamma Region

The Gamma region consists of the Immunoglobulins. This is the area where you will find monoclonal proteins that characterize plasma cell dyscrasias. Note that the IgM migrates closer to the beta region, IgA between beta and gamma peaks, IgG throughout the gamma region.

MGUS

Have a look at a typical SPEP pattern seen in someone with a MGUS.

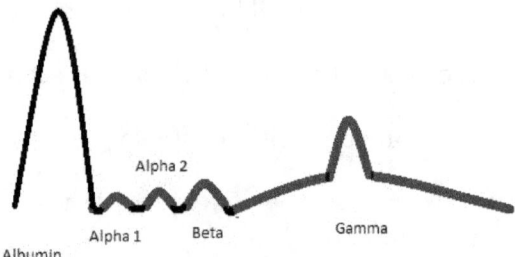

Mononclonal Gammopathy of Undetermined Significance

Albumin

Alpha 1

Alpha 2

Beta

Gamma

Have a look at a typical SPEP pattern seen in someone with a Multiple Myeloma as seen on the next page.

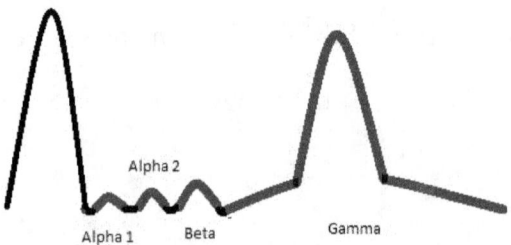

Multiple Myeloma

The SPEP is a Screening Test

The SPEP can provide a quantitative estimate of the concentration of the M-protein.

Immunofixation electrophoresis (IFE) separates the M protein into IgG, IgA, or IgM.

Urine Protein Electrophoresis

UPEP and Urine Immunofixation can be used to test a 24 hour urine collection to detect light chain secretion that is often missed on SPEP because is rapidly excreted in the urine.

Serum Free Light Chains

A Serum Free Light Chains Assay is used to detect low levels of monoclonal free light chains in the serum. It is more sensitive than the UPEP.

MGUS

A monoclonal gammopathy of undetermined significance (MGUS) is characterized by a M-spike is $\leq$3g/dl and <10% plasma cells in bone marrow and lack of end organ damage.

End Organ Damage

End organ damage of plasma cell dyscrasias can be characterized by hypercalcemia with calcium level > 11.5 mg/ dL, renal insufficiency with serum creatinine > 2.0 mg/ dL or estimated creatinine clearance < 40 mL/ min, normochromic normocytic anemia with a hemoglobin value < 10 g/ dL (or a hemoglobin value < 2 g/ dL below the lower limit of normal), and bone lesions (lytic lesions, severe osteopenia, or pathological fractures).

MGUS

MGUS can be divided into 2 categories. (1) lymphoid (or lymphoplasmacytoid) MGUS (2) plasma cell MGUS.

MGUS

About 80-85% of MGUS will be IgG, IgA, IgE. The majority of these are characterized as plasma cell phenotype.

MGUS

Patients with plasma cell MGUS are at risk of progression to multiple myeloma or related plasma cell disorders.

MGUS

About 15-20% of MGUS will secrete IgM.
Most of these are characterized as lymphoid
(lymphoplasmacytoid).

MGUS

Patients with lymphoid MGUS may progress to Waldenström macroglobulinemia, lymphoma, or other malignant lymphoproliferative disorders.

MGUS

We can risk stratify patients with MGUS to determine who is most likely to evolve into a Multiple Myeloma.

MGUS

Global DNA hypomethylation and gene-specific DNA hypermethylation are the most important epigenetic changes that occur during the transformation from MGUS to multiple myeloma.

MGUS

The serum free light chain ratio can be used as a prognostic indicator in patients with MGUS.

Mayo Clinic Risk Stratification MGUS (3 Risk Factors)

(1) High serum M-protein level (> 1.5 g/ dL)

(2) Non-IgG MGUS

(3) An abnormal serum Free Light Chain ratio (defined as < 0.26 or > 1.65)

MGUS Mayo Clinic Risk Stratification

20 year risk of progression to Multiple Myeloma

0 Risk factors- 5%

1 Risk factor- 21%

2 Risk Factors- 37%

3 Risk factors- 58%

Mayo Clinic MGUS Risk Stratification Criteria

In low-risk MGUS patients with no concerning symptoms (anemia or poor renal function), no further initial evaluation is needed. These patients should be followed with SPEP, CBC, calcium, and creatinine at 6 months and, if stable, every 2 to 3 years after that.

MGUS Initial Evaluation with Risk Factors

If any risk factor is present, the patient should be evaluated with baseline bone marrow examination with cytogenetics and FISH studies in addition to bone imaging studies such as skeletal surveys.

MGUS with Risk Factors

Intermediate and high risk MGUS patients should be followed with an SPEP every 6 months for the first year, followed by annual SPEP and routine laboratory tests.

MGUS with Risk Factors

Now let us review the diagnosis of smoldering myeloma.

Smoldering Multiple Myeloma

Smoldering multiple myeloma is defined by patients who have an M-protein concentration $\geq$3 g/dL, 10% and/or more abnormal plasma cells in the bone marrow in the absence of end organ damage (one or more of the following: hypercalcemia, renal failure, anemia, bone lesions).

Smoldering Multiple Myeloma

Patients with smoldering multiple myeloma should undergo baseline bone marrow examination and skeletal survey. The guidelines recommend magnetic resonance imaging (MRI) of the spine and pelvis to detect occult lesions, which, if present, predict for a more rapid progression to multiple myeloma.

Smoldering Myeloma

Mayo Clinic Data estimates the risk of progression from smoldering multiple myeloma to multiple myeloma is 10% per year for the first 5 years, 3% per year for the next 5 years, and 1% for the subsequent 10 years.

Smoldering Myeloma

A randomized study compared zoledronic acid versus surveillance in smoldering multiple myeloma. This study showed a reduced skeletal events in the zoledronic acid arm (55.5% vs surveillance 78.3%). The study found no difference in median time to progression to multiple myeloma.

Mayo Clinic Risk Stratification Smoldering Multiple Myeloma (3 Risk Factors)

(1) High serum M-protein level ($\geq$ 3 g/ dL)

(2) $\geq$ 10% clonal bone marrow plasma cells

(3) An abnormal serum Free Light Chain ratio (defined as < 0.125 or > 8)

Smoldering Myeloma Mayo Clinic Risk Stratification

5 year risk of progression to Multiple Myeloma

1 Risk factor- 25%

2 Risk Factors- 51%

3 Risk factors- 76%

Smoldering Myeloma

Smoldering multiple myeloma patients should have an SPEP and physician evaluation repeated every 2 to 3 months for first year, followed by every 4 to 6 months for another year, with eventual 6 to 12 month evaluations if clinically stable thereafter.

Smoldering Myeloma

Smoldering multiple myeloma is generally not treated outside of clinical trials.

Plasmacytoma

Now let us transition to plasmacytomas.

Plasmacytoma

A plasmacytoma is defined as a malignant plasma cell tumor growing within the soft tissue or within the axial skeleton.

Plasmacytoma

Malignant plasmacytomas can be separated into 2 groups. These are characterized as solitary bone plasmacytomas solitary extramedullary plasmacytomas.

Plasmacytoma

A solitary bone plasmacytoma develops from the plasma cells located in the bone marrow and extramedullary plasmacytoma arises from plasma cells located in mucosal surfaces.

Plasmacytoma

To make the diagnosis of solitary plasmacytoma you must complete a complete evaluation to rule out the presence of systemic disease.

Solitary Bone Plasmacytoma Diagnostic Criteria

(1)Single area of bone destruction by clonal plasma cells (2) Bone marrow plasma cell infiltration not exceeding 5% of all nucleated cells.(3) Absence of osteolytic bone lesions or other tissue involvement (no myeloma). (4) Absence of anemia, hypercalcemia, or renal impairment attributable to myeloma. (5) Low, if present, concentrations of serum or urine monoclonal protein. (6) Preserved levels of uninvolved immunoglobulins.

Extramedullary plasmacytoma Diagnostic criteria

(1)Tissue biopsy showing monoclonal plasma cell histology (2)Bone marrow plasma cell infiltration not exceeding 5% of all nucleated cells (3) Absence of osteolytic bone lesions or other tissue involvement (no evidence of myeloma) (4) Absence of hypercalcemia or renal failure (5) Low or no serum M protein concentration.

Plasmacytoma

Solitary bone plasmacytomas are uncommon
and make up approximately 5% of all of the
plasma cell disorders.

Plasmacytoma

Solitary extramedullary plasmacytomas are less common and represents approximately 3% of all plasma cell disorders.

Plasmacytoma

About 80-90% of extramedullary plasmacytomas presents as a mass found in the aerodigestive tract. The most common location is the tonsils or at the back of the nose. Other disease locations include the nervous system, bladder, thyroid gland (in the neck), breasts, testicles, salivary glands and lymph nodes.

Plasmacytoma

The most common sites for an solitary bone plasmacytoma include the spine and the long bones of the arms and legs. When a solitary plasmacytoma occurs in bone, the first symptoms patients notice are usually pain and tenderness in the affected bone.

Plasmacytoma

Solitary extramedullary plasmacytoma will progress to multiple myeloma in 10-40% of patients at 10 years.

Plasmacytoma

Solitary bone plasmacytoma will progress to multiple myeloma in 50-80% of patients at 10 years.

Plasmacytoma

Solitary bone plasmacytoma rarely involves lymph nodes. Solitary extramedullary plasmacytoma will have lymph node involvement 30%-40% of the time.

Plasmacytoma

Solitary bone plasmacytoma could be considered an intermediate step in the evolution from monoclonal gammopathy of undetermined significance to multiple myeloma.

Plasmacytoma

Patients with solitary bone plasmacytoma who have peripheral polyneuropathy should be evaluated for POEMS syndrome (polyneuropathy, organomegaly, endocrinopathy, M protein, and skin changes).

Plasmacytoma

Solitary osseous plasmacytoma is potentially curable when treated with radiation therapy ($\geq$ 45 Gy) to the involved field.

Plasmacytoma

Extraosseous plasmacytomas are treated with radiation therapy ($\geq$ 45 Gy) to the involved field followed by surgery if necessary.

Multiple Myeloma

Now let us review the diagnosis of multiple myeloma.

Multiple Myeloma

Multiple myeloma is a malignancy of the plasma cells that accounts for 1% of all cancers and 10% of hematological malignancies.

Multiple Myeloma

The CRAB criteria for multiple myeloma are characterized by hypercalcemia, renal failure, anemia or lytic bone lesions.

Staging Multiple Myeloma

ISS Stage I- Serum beta-2 microglobulin is less than 3.5 (mg/L) and the albumin level is 3.5 (g/dL) or greater.

Staging Multiple Myeloma

ISS Stage II- meaning that either: The beta-2 microglobulin level is between 3.5 and 5.5 (with any albumin level), or the albumin is below 3.5 while the beta-2 microglobulin is less than 3.5.

Staging Multiple Myeloma

ISS Stage III- Serum beta-2 microglobulin is 5.5 or greater.

Prognosis Multiple Myeloma

We can sometimes determine poor prognosis by evaluating the multiple myeloma cytogenetics.

Multiple Myeloma Cytogenetics

Poor risk cytogenetic profiles: cytogenetically detected chromosomal 13 or 13q deletion, t(4;14), and del17p; and detection by FISH of t(4;14), t(14;16), and del17p.

Multiple Myeloma Cytogenetics

A translocation between 11 and 14 [t(11;14)] is reported as associated with improved survival.

Multiple Myeloma

Now let us review the multiple myeloma treatment options.

Multiple Myeloma

We must first consider if the patient is a candidate for high-dose therapy and stem cell transplant.

Multiple Myeloma

Advanced age and renal dysfunction are not absolute contraindications to stem cell transplant.

Multiple Myeloma Treatment

Melphalan and Prednisone was the standard of care for treatment of multiple myeloma for more than 3 decades. This combination produces a partial response 40% to 60% of patients, with < 5% comlete response rate, and a progression free survival of approximately 18 months, and overall survival of 2-3 years. Melphalan and prednisone is not used in patients who are candidates for stem cell transplant.

Multiple Myeloma Treatment

We now have many treatment options that are considered superior to melphalan and prednisone.

Multiple Myeloma Treatment for Transplant Candidates

Category 1 treatment options for multiple myeloma patients who are transplant candidates include (1) Bortezomib/dexamethasone (2) Bortezomib/doxorubicin/dexamethasone (3) Bortezomib/doxorubicin/dexamethasone (4) Lenalidomide/dexamethasone.

Multiple Myeloma Treatment for Transplant Candidates

Category 2a treatment options for multiple myeloma patients who are transplant candidates include (1) Bortezomib/lenalidomide/dexamethasone (2) Cyclophosphamide/bortezomib/dexamethasone.

Multiple Myeloma Treatment for Transplant Candidates

Category 2b treatment options for multiple myeloma patients who are transplant candidates include (1) Thalidomide/Dexamethasone (2) Single-Agent Dexamethasone (3) Liposomal doxorubicin/vincristine/dexamethasone.

Multiple Myeloma Treatment for Patients who are not Transplant Candidates

Category 1a treatment options for multiple myeloma patients who are not transplant candidates include (1) Melphalan/prednisone/thalidomide (2) Melphalan/prednisone/bortezomib (3) Melphalan/prednisone/lenalidomide (4) Lenalidomide/Low-dose dexamethasone.

Multiple Myeloma Treatment for Patients who are not Transplant Candidates

Category 2a treatment options for multiple myeloma patients who are not transplant candidates include (1) Bortezomib/dexamethasone (2) Melphalan and prednisone.

Multiple Myeloma Treatment for Patients who are not Transplant Candidates

Category 2b treatment options for multiple myeloma patients who are not transplant candidates include (1) Bortezomib/dexamethasone (2) Melphalan and prednisone (3) Thalidomide/dexamethasone, (4) Single-agent dexamethasone, (5) Liposomal doxorubicin/vincristine/dexamethasone (6) VAD.

Multiple Myeloma Treatment

Lenalidomide and high-dose dexamethasone was compared with lenalidomide and low-dose dexamethasone in newly diagnosed multiple myeloma patients. Lenalidomide and high-dose dexamethasone was associated with a higher overall response rate than lenalidomide and low-dose dexamethasone (79% vs 68%) but the 1-year overall survival was superior for low-dose dexamethasone. A survival benefit was observed with lenalidomide and low-dose dexamethasone regimen in patients more than 65 years of age.

Multiple Myeloma

Since there are several possible options for
treating multiple myeloma. Let us look at a
few scenarios.

Multiple Myeloma

Alkylating containing regimens such as Velcade, Melphalan and Prednisone or Melphalan, Prednisone can be used to treat elderly patients with good performance status.

Multiple Myeloma

Bortezomib/Doxorubicin/Dexamethasone is a viable treatment option for patients with deletion of chromosome 13q.

Multiple Myeloma

Patients with renal failure can be treated with full dose bortezomib or thalidomide. If treated with lenalidomide, dose adjustments based on creatinine clearance must be made.

Multiple Myeloma

Bortezomib based combination chemotherapy is less thrombogenic and may be a good option for patients with a history of thrombembolism.

Multiple Myeloma

Melphalan, Prednisone, and Revlimid, or
Revlimid and Dexamethasone, or
bendamustine plus prednisone would be a
good choice for patients with preexisting
neuropathy because these are associated with
less neurotoxicity.

Multiple Myeloma

A bortezomib-containing regimen is a good choice for up-front treatment. In patients with del(13) or t(4;14) cytogenetic abnormality.

Multiple Myeloma

The combination of (Melphalan, Prednisone, and Thalidomide), (Velcade, Melphalan and Prednisone) (Melphalan, Prednisone, and Revlimid), and (Lenalidomide and dexamethasone) provides are all options for first line treatment in elderly patients.

Multiple Myeloma

Multiple myeloma treatment can be tailored for patients based on potential treatment toxicity.

Multiple Myeloma

The risk of herpes zoster activation in patients treated with bortezomib can be reduced with the use of prophylactic acyclovir.

Multiple Myeloma

The most common toxicities associated with
thalidomide/dexamethasone were venous
thromboembolism (15.3%).

Multiple Myeloma

Anticoagulation is used in patients treated with Melphalan/Prednisone/Thalidomide because of the risk of DVT with thalidomide-based therapy.

Multiple Myeloma Stem Cell Transplant

Many patients will be a candidate for a
stem cell transplant.

Multiple Myeloma Stem Cell Transplant

A single autologous stem cell transplant in combination with high dose chemotherapy is a treatment approach for multiple myeloma that can lead to a durable response. Tandem autologous stem cell transplants are reserved for patients who do not have a very good partial response to a Single autologous HSCT.

Multiple Myeloma Stem Cell Transplant

Selection for autologous stem cell transplant in the United States takes into consideration the age of the patient in conjunction with performance status, frailty, and comorbidities (including cardiac, pulmonary, hepatic, and renal function).

Multiple Myeloma Stem Cell Transplant

Hematopoietic cell transplant comorbidity index calculates a score based on other common medical problems and is predictive of survival after autologous hematopoietic cell transplantation in multiple myeloma.

Multiple Myeloma Stem Cell Transplant

Autologous stem cell transplants are common, however allogeneic stem cell transplant is not clearly established as a standard treatment approach for most multiple myeloma patients.

Multiple Myeloma Stem Cell Transplant

Double or tandem autologous HSCT has been shown to be superior to single autologous HSCT in patients who do not attain at least a very good partial response.

Multiple Myeloma Stem Cell Transplant

It is not certain whether tandem autologous HSCT up-front is superior to a single transplantation followed by second autologous HSCT after disease progression.

Multiple Myeloma Stem Cell Transplant

Three collection approaches include chemotherapy mobilization with growth factor support (G-CSF), G-CSF with plerixafor, or G-CSF alone.

Multiple Myeloma Stem Cell Transplant

Autologous stem cell transplant preparation regimens generally consist of dose-intensive regimens high-dose melphalan.

Multiple Myeloma Stem Cell Transplant

Maintenance therapy after autologous stem cell transplant for multiple myeloma has been shown beneficial.

Multiple Myeloma Stem Cell Transplant

Thalidomide maintenance after autologous stem cell transplant improves PFS and OS in some studies but not in high-risk disease.

Multiple Myeloma Stem Cell Transplant

Most patients cannot stay on maintenance therapy with thalidomide even in low doses because of neuropathic side effects.

Multiple Myeloma Stem Cell Transplant

Lenalidomide maintenance after autologous HSCT has reported shown to improve PFS or time to progression.

Multiple Myeloma Stem Cell Transplant

Bortezomib maintenance after autologous HSCT has been reported to improve both PFS and OS.

This concludes MGUS, Plasmacytoma and
Multiple Myeloma: Fast Focus Study Guide

Search Amazon Kindle books to find other study
guides written by

JT Thomas, MD

Internal Medicine Study Guide

Hematology Study Guide

Medical Oncology Study Guide

Cardiology Study Guide

Multiple Myeloma Study Guide

Differential Diagnosis Study Guide

Rheumatology Study Guide

Cancer Study Guide